TERMINAL
CANCER
—— IS A ——
MISDIAGNOSIS

Discover A Palliative Care Alternative
Medicine You Can Survive

DANNY CARROLL

Praise for
Terminal Cancer Is a Misdiagnosis

"What exactly is Cancer? That is the question. If you want to revolutionize your whole concept of what cancer really is, then you should read this book. The message is one of hope. It is like a silver thread that can be seen and felt throughout. It makes us aware of our erroneous, default belief: that illness must originate with a pathogen, or something that we may have done or consumed…As a counselor, I am very interested in trauma, as well as how it impacts, and is impacted by our emotions. Reading what Dr. Hamer discovered — that intricate link between emotional trauma and cancer — validated everything that I intrinsically knew and had observed in my own practice."

—Tessa Anthia John Guerra, Licensed Psychologist & Psychotherapist

"Danny Carroll's wonderful book, *Terminal Cancer Is a Misdiagnosis,* is essential reading for anyone who is living with cancer or any life-threatening illness. The body can heal when your head and your heart find their way home. Danny Carroll reveals the dynamics behind this phenomenon in a clear, articulate manner, making this book a treasure and, yes, a potential lifesaver for those who read it!"

— CJ Scarlet, author of *Heroic Parenting* and *Badass Parenting*

"This book has a big and compelling title that sets the expectation bar high. Yet, it is the result of a determined quest by the author over many, many years, to reveal a solution to the most dreaded illnesses of mankind. His exploration revealed the work of a great, yet controversial maverick in the field of cancer treatment…Furthermore, I am gratified that this work squares with my own personal experience with cancer. Of the half-dozen of my loved ones who died due to this scourge of an illness, all had suffered traumatic life events that preceded their cancer diagnoses. For me, it is now clear that this spirit-rending trauma was the prelude to their cancer."

—T. L. Needham, award-winning author of *When I Was a Child*

ISBN:

Issued in print and electronic formats.

ISBN 978-1-915838-00-1 TCIAM (eBook)
ISBN 978-1-915838-01-8 TCIAM (Paperback)
ISBN 978-1-915838-02-5 TCIAM (Hardback)
ISBN 978-1-915838-03-2 TCIAM (Audiobook)

Disclaimer:

Please note: The author of this book is not a medical doctor. The information contained in this book is for educational purposes only. All effort has been made to present accurate, up-to-date, complete, and reliable information. No warranties of any kind are stated or implied. Readers acknowledge that the author is not engaging in the rendering of medical, legal, financial, or professional advice. Please consult a licensed professional before attempting any techniques outlined in this book.

Under no circumstances will any legal responsibility be held against the publisher or author for any damages, reparations, or monetary loss due to the information contained within this book, neither directly nor indirectly. The content within this book has been derived from multiple sources, including details of the author's own healing experiences.

By reading this book, the reader agrees that under no circumstances will the author be held responsible for any losses, direct or indirect, which are incurred as a result of implementing the information contained in this book, including, but not limited to, errors, omissions, or inaccuracies. You are responsible for your own choices, actions, and results.

Dedication

This book is dedicated to Parveen Aga, Dr. Ryke Geerd Hamer, and Helmut Pilhar.

In my ignorance and overenthusiasm, I unknowingly made a significant contribution to Parveen Aga's life ending long before it was her time to move on. Her death from the aftereffects of chemotherapy inspired me to search to the ends of the earth to find a better solution to cancer.

I sadly did not get to meet Dr. Hamer before he died in 2017. Without a doubt, he was the greatest medical mind in the history of mankind. He singlehandedly unraveled the biological code and then spent the rest of his life being persecuted for his medical discoveries.

Helmut Pilhar was Dr. Hamer's chosen lecturer to spread Germanic Healing Knowledge. Helmut was the tip of the spear and dedicated his life to teaching GHk. He sadly passed away on 31 August 2022.

May their souls rest in eternal peace.

CONTENTS

INTRODUCTION

*P*eople often ask me, "How many people have you healed from cancer?"

My answer is always, "One person: myself." Healing others is impossible; it is only possible to heal yourself.

The fact that you are responsible for your own health, or the lack thereof, may be shocking to those who have allowed others, out of fear, to dictate their medical decisions (often ignoring their own instincts). For others, it is empowering.

You are not a victim. You can heal.

The major drawback to today's medical paradigm is that it is a system of symptom treatment. For most health problems, drugs are prescribed to counteract the symptoms. Anyone who has worked in an organization, whether it is a business, charity, or an NGO, will be familiar with the following concept: If you only deal with the symptoms of a problem, and not the root cause, it will return repeatedly.

Today, this is what we are doing with our health, and it is why we end up with chronic health issues. This is good if you are in the business of selling pharmaceuticals. It is not so good if you are the consumer.

In the last report I read, the average cancer patient in America was worth $1 million to the medical system.[1] Money corrupts... and with this type of money to be made, there is a strong incentive to diagnose as many people as possible with cancer. I would love to be wrong about this. Unfortunately, my years of experience leave me in a position where I can draw no other logical conclusion.

Watching my dear friend die needlessly from the aftereffects of chemotherapy is what led me on my 17-year journey searching for the holy grail of health and wellness. Studying both mainstream and alternative medicine modalities, the fundamental issue I discovered was that they are ALL systems of symptomatic treatment. None address the "cause" of the problem.

Then I discovered the scientific body of knowledge, Dr. Ryke Geerd Hamer's Germanic New Medicine/Germanische Heilkunde. This is loosely translated in English as Germanic Healing Knowledge.

In Dr. Hamer's medical science, the Germanic Healing Knowledge, there is no such diagnosis as terminal cancer.

Just because a doctor has given you a terminal diagnosis does not mean it is the end of the road. They are still interpreting your symptoms through centuries of medical dogma — and the commercial interests that have been increasingly exploiting healthcare for profit since the late 1800s. A large hospital can give you the best organ-level diagnosis of your symptoms. Unfortunately, the doctors working there are only allowed to manage those symptoms with drugs, surgery, and radiation.

As a member of a private, professional organization, your doctor would be risking their license if they attempted to address the root cause(s) of the issues affecting your health. Dr. Hamer found this out the hard way. Today, however, an experienced Germanic Healing Knowledge consultant, operating outside of this monopoly, can help you navigate this revolutionary understanding of how our biology functions and get to the root cause of your disease.

If you have been given a diagnosis of an incurable, terminal cancer by a medical doctor and sent home to die, read this book to discover:

- Why many diagnoses are incorrect.

- A six-year cancer research study that resulted in an 85% survival rate for cancer patients who refused standard medical treatment.

- How to switch off excruciating pain triggered by a terminal diagnosis.

- Principles and healing protocols that apply to all cancer diagnoses, regardless of stage.

- How Germanic Healing Knowledge therapy is the only exception I have ever found to the rule, "If it's too good to be true, it probably is."

- Music therapy to place your disease on hold while you address its emotional origins.

Additionally, sign up at my website **danny-carroll.com** to receive:

- A step-by-step resource guide, including a list of Germanic Healing Knowledge (GHk) consultants and educational materials. Both are highly recommended to embark on what may be the most extraordinary journey of your life — to fully recover your health.

- A 400+ page e-book with over 500 case study examples detailing the "cause" of nearly every known disease.

- A one-year course of daily, 6–7-minute MP3 Germanic Healing Knowledge classes.

- The monthly digest, *The Healing Tribune - The Cause of Disease Made Simple.* This digest explores the cause and treatments for disease through both a Conventional Medicine and a Germanic Healing Knowledge perspective. Readers decide which is more compelling. There will be 500+ digest copies written over time, one for each disease.

CHAPTER 1
MY JOURNEY OF DISCOVERY

*I*n the mid 2000s, a close friend and colleague of mine named Parveen Aga was diagnosed with cancer. Without health insurance or money for her cancer treatments, I ran a marathon to raise money from friends and well-wishers. She was delighted. Still, even though the doctors said she was sick, Parveen looked perfectly fine to me…until she started her chemotherapy treatments.

Parveen would text me from the hospital saying, "I have no idea what these doctors are doing, but it feels like they are putting poison in my veins." At the time, I did not know any better. In my eagerness to help, I strongly encouraged her to keep taking the treatments.

After three rounds of chemo, she was dead.

I was devastated and haunted by the thought that by both financing and ensuring her compliance with the treatment, I had played a significant role in Parveen's death. She had been very dear and close to me, and I felt responsible for her leaving this earth long before it was her time. She was only in her early sixties. That was the moment when I vowed to devote my life to finding a better solution to cancer.

The Seventeen-Year Search Begins

I began my research into every mainstream and alternate healing therapy I could find, from nutritional and emotional healing to energy and spiritual healing. As an analytical, process-type person, I need to understand the problem and what causes it. If someone proposes a solution, how does it work? If there is one thing that was drilled into my head over many long years of business consulting, it is input-process-output.

Soon, the problem I faced with every healing modality I studied was that when two people with the same diagnosis were treated with the same protocol, one might live while the other died. Despite my insatiable curiosity, no amount of research could explain why this was consistently the case. After years of searching, I could not say with confidence that I had found definitive answers to any health challenges — and especially not for something like cancer.

It took my own health crisis to discover the answer.

The Mind-Body Connection

In 2012, the muscles in my entire body had been riddled with golf-ball-sized knots. I am a passionate marathon runner and could barely walk during this period, forget running. I spent six months in physiotherapy having them ironed out of my muscles — an extremely painful process. Still, two days after the treatment, they would return with a vengeance. It was like an excruciating merry-go-round.

At the time, I was facing a unique challenge in my life. My girlfriend was on a fixed, two-year posting in my hometown, and her next posting was going to be 10,000 miles away — a 40-hour journey from where I lived. We had planned to end our relationship when she left, but there was a problem: we had become soul mates. At the end of November of that year, we agreed that instead of breaking up, we would continue with a long-distance relationship and see if it fizzled out naturally.

When I woke up the next morning, the knots that had riddled my body for the last six months had all disappeared! I had no idea how it had happened. The only difference between Friday night and Saturday morning was that I had resolved the conflict over ending the relationship with my girlfriend.

With no more physical complaints, I returned to marathon training. My normal training period for a full marathon was at least three to four months, and the Mumbai Marathon was one month away. Without a single cramp or injury, I finished the 42-kilometer marathon 11 minutes short of my personal best time. This cathartic experience helped me understand the power of the mind and how it can heal or hinder us.

By then, I had already dedicated seven years of my free time to working with late-stage, terminally ill cancer patients (and I continue to do so). As I mentioned in the dedication, this was a result of my friend's death, as well as a part of my Corporate Social Responsibility commitment. Living in India, you do not have to go far to find people in need of help. I tried various complementary and alternative treatments with cancer patients, still looking for that ever-elusive way to resolve their suffering.

After experiencing how my mind had crippled me with golf-ball-sized knots — and how they had disappeared overnight — I had a strong suspicion that there must be some relationship between the mind and cancer.

I had planned to take a few years off and make this the focus of a PhD. I wanted to study this phenomenon and understand the possibility of a mind-cancer connection. While looking for a university that would support my PhD proposal, I came across a German medical doctor named Ryke Geerd Hamer. Reports indicated that he was achieving success rates of over 90%, healing late-stage cancer patients with a form of mind-body healing.

Since then, I have spent the last ten years studying the biological science discovered by Dr. Hamer, a conventionally trained and licensed medical doctor. He referred to his discoveries as Germanic New Medicine (GNM), but he later renamed it *Germanische Heilkunde,* which loosely translates into English as Germanic Healing Knowledge (GHk).

Dr. Hamer's findings are extraordinary.

CHAPTER 2
DR. HAMER'S JOURNEY OF DISCOVERY

*D*r. Hamer began studying the mind-cancer connection in 1978, after a diagnosis of testicular and abdominal cancer. Informed that his entire abdomen was full of metastases, he was given a 1% chance of survival. The diagnosis came two months after the death of his 19-year-old son, Dirk, who had been accidentally shot on the island of Cavallo by the Italian crown prince, Prince Victor Emmanuel of Savoy.

After 17 surgeries and months of suffering, Dirk died in his father's arms. A healthy man his entire life, Dr. Hamer could not help thinking that there must be some link between his devastation over his son's death and his own cancer diagnosis. Unlike the traditional belief that his "disease" was a random growth in his testicle, an abnormal, fast-growing, and uncontrollable (malignant) tumor with no specific cause, Dr. Hamer would later conclude that his cancer was a biological program triggered by the untimely death of his son.

Dr. Hamer underwent surgery for testicular cancer and metastases in his abdomen but refused chemotherapy and radiation (as I understand over 90% of medical doctors do when they have a cancer diagnosis themselves). Once recovered, he was in the perfect position to follow up on his hypothesis. Dr. Hamer was an internal medicine specialist and, at the time, the chief resident at a gynecological cancer research center affiliated with the Munich University Clinic. There, he carried out in-depth interviews with 200 confirmed cancer patients to discern whether they had suffered from similarly distressing events before their diagnoses.

Without exception, all the cancer patients had experienced some type of trauma.

Dr. Hamer concluded that cancer is a "survival" biological program. When we face an unexpected, distressing event/ emotional trauma, the biological program we call cancer is triggered to increase (or decrease) the capacity of a specific organ. This helps us overcome the problem and ensure our survival.

In Dr. Hamer's case, his son died. Tissue was added to his testicle to increase his capacity to produce testosterone and sperm. The biological purpose was to increase his ability to get his wife pregnant to replace the child he just lost.

The Iron Rule of Cancer

Over time, Dr. Hamer worked with over 50,000 patients to complete his medical research findings and establish what is now known as The Iron Rule of Cancer. It states that cancer can only be caused by what he called a biological conflict shock that catches you on the wrong foot, is dramatic, isolates you in your predicament, and affects you on three levels: the psyche, the brain, and the organ.

Perceived in the psyche, this unexpected distress or trauma leaves a physical impression, a set of target rings on the relay in the brain that is associated with a specific organ, and starts a physiological process — an adaptation — in the organ itself. These foci can be seen on the brain via a computed tomography (CT) scan.

In time, Dr. Hamer could determine someone's entire medical history from a brain CT scan.

In 1991, Dr. Hamer presented his medical discoveries to a group of doctors. One of the attending physicians gave Dr. Hamer a brain CT scan of one of the patients in the hospital. He asked Dr. Hamer if he could diagnose the health issues the patient was facing by only reading the brain scan. Dr. Hamer had no prior knowledge of the patient's medical history.

After a lecture I gave in Vienna in May 1991, a doctor handed me a brain computed tomogram of a patient and asked me to disclose the person's organic state, and to which conflict it belonged. There were twenty colleagues present, including some radiologists and CT specialists. Of the three levels (psyche, brain, organ), I had only the brain level in front of me.

From these brain CT scans, I was able to diagnose a fresh bleeding bladder carcinoma in the healing phase, an old prostate carcinoma, diabetes, an old lung carcinoma, and a sensory paralysis of a specific area in the body, and, of course, the corresponding conflicts.

The doctor stood up and congratulated me. "Five diagnoses and five hits. That is exactly what the patient has, and you were even able to differentiate what he has now and what he had before. Fantastic!"

One of the radiologists told me, "I am convinced of your method. How could you have guessed the fresh bleeding bladder carcinoma? I could find nothing in the CT scan but now that you have shown us the relay, I can understand the findings."[1]

Ignoring the Evidence

Dr. Hamer presented his initial findings on the connection between biological conflicts and cancer as a post-doctoral thesis to the University of Tübingen (where he had graduated medical school). However, the university's review committee immediately rejected his work without even evaluating it.

What is more, after Dr. Hamer shared his findings with his Bavarian colleagues, he was quickly given an ultimatum: either repudiate his findings or face dismissal. Refusing to retract his medical discoveries, he was summarily dismissed. Even though German law requires universities to review all post-doctoral submissions, the University of Tübingen later admitted in court that they never made any attempt to confirm Dr. Hamer's medical discoveries. When the presiding judge asked university representatives why they had defied a court order, they replied:

"We do not want to know whether Dr. Hamer is right or not."

Even when his medical license was revoked and a court-ordered injunction was issued against him, Dr. Hamer never stopped consulting the desperately ill. In 1993, Dr. Hamer was prosecuted in Austria for practicing medicine without a license. The Public Prosecutor's Office of Neustadt subpoenaed the medical records of over 6,500 of Dr. Hamer's patients (many of whom had been previously diagnosed as terminally ill).

After tracking down these patients in person to find out their current state of health, the prosecution had to admit in court that over 6,000, or over 90%, were not only alive, but had fully recovered their health. Dr. Hamer was subsequently convicted for practicing medicine without a license.

After two different prison sentences that totaled two and a half years, the courts in Germany and France had to conclude that Dr. Hamer had been unjustly prosecuted, and he was released. One must stop and question why someone who successfully helped thousands of cancer patients to fully recover their health, lost his medical license and was imprisoned. The answer is simple: Dr. Hamer defied the standard treatment protocol and refused to prescribe chemotherapy.

But it did not end there. In the following decades, Dr. Hamer was categorically vilified on television programs in German-speaking countries, and dozens of attempts were made to have him declared mentally insane and institutionalized. He even survived violent attacks on his life. Now you understand why the world has not heard of Dr. Hamer's breakthrough medical discoveries.

The End of Conventional Medicine?

Dr. Hamer estimated that were his medical discoveries allowed to surface and become accepted in mainstream society, 95% of today's conventional medicine treatment protocols and procedures would be obsolete. People would heal themselves so a healthcare system would no longer be required.

Very few people have been exposed to this information — and even fewer have taken the time to investigate it for themselves. I consider myself lucky. It took me seven years of searching for better cancer solutions before I even found Dr. Hamer. Sadly, he passed away in July of 2017. A truly extraordinary man, Dr. Hamer's medical discoveries are a great gift to humanity.

Humanity, however, just needs to discover and understand this gift for themselves…and there is no better time than when the doctors give you a death sentence and send you home to die.

CHAPTER 3
SWITCH OFF CANCER

*W*e have been deeply conditioned by the conventional medicine system to think that all diseases are caused by outside factors. These factors include smoking, viruses, industrial chemicals, bad lifestyle habits, radiation from mobile phones and towers, etc. The idea that our illnesses are caused by distressing conflict shocks/traumas (except for poisoning, injuries from accidents, and nutritional deficiency diseases, e.g., scurvy through a lack of vitamin C), is not an easy pill to swallow — excuse the pun.

Dr. Hamer discovered that cancer and cancer-equivalent diseases, e.g. heart attacks, multiple sclerosis, etc., have components that I term, "The Bioswitch Theory." The following apply to all the conditions we call diseases:

- On switch
- Off switch
- Biological significance/purpose

On Switch

The on switch is found in the part of your subconscious mind we call the psyche. It involves your senses, brain, and nervous system, and it is always aware and alert for danger.

According to Dr. Hamer, the on switch is triggered by an unexpected, distressing event that catches you on the wrong foot. It is highly acute and dramatic, and isolates you in your predicament. Dr. Hamer experienced this unexpected biological conflict shock when his son Dirk died in his arms. This started his testicular and stomach cancer programs to run.

When we experience this unexpected shock, in a split second, it simultaneously affects the psyche, brain, and corresponding organ, like an electric shock. This triggers the start of the first phase of disease Dr. Hamer named the "conflict active" phase. Constantly thinking about the problem, you will often wake up at 3 AM to have more waking hours to solve the conflict. Symptoms include cold hands and feet as blood flow to your extremities is reduced, diminished appetite, and weight loss.

At the organ level, physiological changes are triggered to change the organs' capacity to help you solve the problem. This includes either adding tissue (a tumor), removing tissue (bone osteolysis, ulceration), or functional loss or enhancement (high or low blood sugar or thyroxin, short-term memory loss, paralysis, etc.).

An easy way to understand the concept of tissue being added and removed is to look at a woman's menstrual cycle. In the first half of a woman's cycle, tissue is added to the walls of the uterus so that it will be prepared for a fertilized egg to implant should she become pregnant. If she does not get pregnant, the extra tissue is removed via bleeding.

The area of the brain and organs affected is determined by the nature and content of the conflict. One example are the lungs. If you have a challenge to your territory (your territory is anything important to you), the bronchi in your lungs and coronary arteries are widened by removing tissue to give you a greater capacity to take in oxygen and get blood to your heart. This serves to send more oxygen to the muscles to help you defend your territory. In our evolutionary development, and in animals to this day, this could be a fight to the death.

Off Switch

There are actually two off switches. The first is a practical resolution of the biological conflict. The best way to switch off a biological program is through a real-life resolution to the conflict that triggered it. Dr. Hamer's sudden and tragic loss of his son led to the development of his testicular cancer. Logically, he later determined that this type of cancer is caused by the conflict of suffering a profound loss.

The biological purpose of a testicular teratoma tumor was to increase his testosterone and sperm production to make him more fertile. If Dr. Hamer had fathered another child, the purpose of that specific biological program would have been achieved and the active program (i.e., the "cancer" or addition of tissue) would have switched off naturally. However, real-life solutions to conflicts are not always possible. Dr. Hamer's son was 19 when he died, and his wife was already past her child-bearing years. Nature, unfortunately, does not factor in the impracticalities built into our modern, civilized culture.

Dr. Hamer discovered that while a biological program is running on autopilot below your level of waking consciousness, when you consciously recall the traumatic event and connect it to the symptoms you are experiencing, you can switch off a disease like a light switch. This is the second off switch.

This is a key part to the Bioswitch Theory, although there is a catch to this off switch: Reminders or "tracks" of the original trauma in your psyche can switch the program back on again. You may have to keep switching it off repeatedly. Programs are only permanently turned off when there is no possibility of it turning on again. No conflict = no problem.

Most physical symptoms are experienced in the second phase, AFTER the conflict is resolved and the switch is turned off. This healing, or repair phase, is accompanied by inflammation, swelling, and pain as the body naturally returns to normal, a state known as homeostasis.

Biological Significance/Purpose

Every "biological program," as Dr. Hamer preferred to call a disease, has a purpose. Once that purpose has been fulfilled, the nervous system switches to the repair phase, which is characterized by parasympathetic (vagotonic) nervous system activity. This is what we commonly consider illness.

The first phase, or conflict-active phase, often proceeds with little or no physical discomfort (unless it has gone on for so long that cell growth compromises other internal organs' functions or becomes otherwise noticeable). The second phase, the healing or repair phase, is usually when someone goes to the doctor with symptoms and an illness or a disease is diagnosed. However, once the repair phase is finished, the entire biological program's job is over, and this two-phase process ends. You are now back to full health and possibly stronger than before.

You have no doubt heard about "spontaneous remissions" with many cancers, including "terminal" cancers. What has in fact happened is that the conflict causing the biological program has been resolved. The repair phase is complete and the body returns to homeostasis. These "miracles" are perfectly natural but a phenomenon that conventional medicine still struggles to explain.

As mentioned earlier, the golf-ball-sized knots in my muscles had the biological purpose of slowing me down from going in the wrong direction in life. I was planning to end the relationship with my soul mate. As soon as I resolved that conflict, by agreeing not to prematurely terminate our relationship, the knots disappeared overnight. That amazing woman is now my beautiful wife. Nature knows best.

Gaining Conviction in Dr. Hamer's Discoveries

As a skeptical person, I need to experience things for myself. I never believe what I read until I have personally tested ideas. There is no other way to gain conviction, and I strongly recommend you take a similar approach. As the years passed after my cathartic healing experience, I followed Dr. Hamer's scientific chart to switch off some of the other disease symptoms (biological programs running) in my body.

Thus far, I have switched off:

- 15 years of irritable bowel syndrome/ulcerative colitis.

- Lactose intolerance: After going vegan to test a nutrition hypothesis for cancer, I was lactose intolerant for five years.

- Eczema/Psoriasis.

- Recurring disc pain in my lower back: I suffered for 15 years and spent weeks and even months working from my bedroom floor.

- Ear and sinus infections.

- A cerebellum constellation: In short, this condition is caused by an attack conflict, and it leaves you emotionally numb and void.

- A loss conflict that had been running for 20 years: It had reduced my left testicle to half its original size (testicular seminoma Leydig cell cancer).

In 2019, I had cancer in my jaw. I finally worked out that it had been triggered by a five-second disagreement with my wife, which made the conflict incredibly difficult to locate. By the time I was able to switch off the cancer program, all my teeth had fallen out on one side of my mouth. I had five hours of reconstructive surgery, including a bone graft, to rebuild the jaw and replace my teeth.

I took one pain killer at the time of the oral surgery and another in the evening. After that, I "switched off" the pain from the surgery and did not need to take any more. It was a truly mind-blowing experience. This was the first time I tried to switch off pain from physical trauma — oral surgery. Previously, I had only turned off pain that had come from the distress following a biological conflict shock.

Pain has a biological purpose of stopping you from using that part of the body so it has the time, space, and energy to heal. When you cut your finger, if you don't use it, you won't feel any pain. As soon as you start using your finger, it will start throbbing. It's nature's way of telling you the finger needs to heal.

I had no teeth so I couldn't use that side of my mouth to chew. I said to my subconscious mind, "I have no teeth so I will not use that side of my mouth to eat. I will give it the time, space and energy to heal. Please switch off the pain. "The pain and throbbing from the surgery stopped immediately!

Whenever food accidentally went to the side of my mouth where I had the surgery, the pain would restart with a vengeance. I apologized to my subconscious mind for the error and struck the deal again. The pain switched off again. For my jaw to recover from the surgery, I slept 20 hours a day for three weeks without pain. The 35 stitches were then removed and my jaw had healed.

Testing the Science

If you want to test this medical science for yourself, think intensely about something you dislike, something in your life that really stinks or sucks. Shortly after you stop, your nose will start running. A runny nose is caused by a "stink conflict." Now, say to your subconscious mind, "I know my nose is running because I was just thinking intensely about something I hate (fill in what you were thinking about). Please switch off my runny nose."

What happened to your runny nose?

If there is a problem in your life that you have been biting your tongue and not talking about, gather the courage to express how you feel. Soon after, your tongue will become hypersensitive, and you will get painful ulcers on the tongue! Now follow the same exercise with your tongue. Say to yourself, "I know my tongue is sore because I was biting my tongue about (fill in the blanks), and I gained the courage to speak my mind."

The level of importance of the issue, and amount of time it takes to finally say how you feel, determines whether you down-grade the pain on the tongue or switch it off completely. The longer you withhold the truth about a critical issue, and the stronger your feelings are about it, the longer it will take the pain to reduce and the ulcer to heal.

Congratulations; you have just learned a way to switch biological programs ("illnesses") on and off.

Once you have personal experience of how this medical science works, every subsequent healing experience increases your conviction.

It is the Holy Grail of health and wellness.

This approach involves you taking responsibility for your own health and is much less convenient than outsourcing your health to your doctor and taking various drugs to solve all your problems. However, I have found that this truth pill becomes much easier to swallow after medical doctors send someone home to die, telling them that nothing else can be done. It does not need to be the end of the road…if you choose it not to be.

CHAPTER 4
WHAT IS CANCER?

*A*ccording to conventional medicine, cancer is a disease caused by the uncontrolled growth of abnormal cells in the body that can form tumors and spread to other organs in a process called metastasis. If cells are multiplying in what doctors consider to be an abnormal and uncontrollable way, the cancer is said to be malignant. If a tumor is not growing and multiplying, it is benign.

Dr. Hamer's observations led him to a vastly different understanding of cancer. He concluded that cancer is a natural, Significant Biological Special Program (SBS) that serves a biological purpose and is a critical part of nature's survival biological program. Dr. Hamer's belief was that when we face an unexpected, distressing event/trauma, the biological program we call cancer is triggered to increase (or decrease) the capacity of a specific organ, to help us overcome the problem.

Dr. Hamer spent 39 years working with over 50,000 patients and mapped out the biological conflicts/traumas that cause all diseases known to man. They are recorded in the Scientific Chart of Germanic New Medicine.[1] All his research was done with empirical cases using the latest medical diagnostic technology. Each case was verified in the psyche, brain, and organ.

Once you understand the basic biological purpose of organ-specific cancer programs, you can verify these phenomena for yourself. Liver cancer is one example.

Liver Cancer and the Starvation Conflict

The main tissue of the liver is called liver parenchyma. Doctors believe that liver parenchyma primarily becomes diseased because of alcohol poisoning. According to Dr. Hamer, liver parenchyma responds to what he described as a starvation conflict.

What doctors fail to consider, and what is easily observable if you have ever known an alcoholic, is that many have erratic eating habits. As their addiction worsens, they frequently skip meals in favor of alcohol. Their disease affects their ability to feel hunger, and many are at risk of malnutrition. Liver cancer is not caused by heavy drinking, but instead by a starvation conflict.[2]

The liver has many functions, but one of the key functions is producing digestive enzymes. If the body is battling starvation, the liver will grow additional tissue. The biological purpose is to increase the production of digestive enzymes so that you can better digest your body's own tissue reserves and survive. When the threat has passed, the liver will naturally revert to its original size and capacity.

Let us compare health statistics for liver cancer in Africa versus the West. In the West, liver cancer typically makes up 1–2% of the total cancer cases diagnosed. In places like Africa, however, where people are starving to death, the rates of liver cancer (as the percent of total cancer cases diagnosed) ranges between 8% and 10%.[3] Large segments of the population in many African countries have little or no money to feed themselves, much less buy alcohol. Liver cancer is one of the primary cancer diagnoses because people are starving.

Liver cancer is diagnosed as one of the most frequent forms of metastatic or secondary cancers. Is it possible that continuous vomiting from chemotherapy poison leads the psyche to conclude that the body is starving to death and thus increases the size and capacity of the liver to prolong survival?

Lung Cancer and Fear-of-Death Conflict

The common belief is that smoking causes lung cancer. According to Dr. Hamer's research, lung cancer (of the alveoli, not the bronchi, goblet cells, or bronchial musculature) is caused by a fear-of-death conflict.

The alveoli make up the bulk of the lungs, where the actual taking in of oxygen and releasing of carbon dioxide occur. Since oxygen is critical for life, when we are unexpectedly confronted with the possibility of dying, the lung(s) respond by increasing our capacity to process oxygen. Our organism wants to keep us alive. This additional buildup of alveoli cells is what doctors diagnose as lung cancer.

According to Dr. Hamer's research findings, the alveoli are affected by a fear-of-death for self or a loved one. Imagine a medical doctor saying, "You have cancer. Without surgery and an immediate start of chemotherapy, you will be dead in a year." Would it be possible that your fear of death triggers cancer in your lungs? Could the resulting diagnosis of metastatic lung cancer be then caused by the doctor's prognosis (outlook)?

When a longstanding fear-of-death conflict is resolved, this extra capacity built up in the lung(s) is then broken down by tuberculosis (TB) mycobacteria (if they have not already been exterminated by heavy doses of antibiotics) and coughed up — an unpleasant, yet effective process.

TB mycobacteria are the body's natural mechanism for removing the extra tissue added during a conflict. These tubercular mycobacteria have an important biological purpose and play a critical role in our lungs' healing process, one that has been terribly misunderstood by the medical system. If the TB microbacteria have been destroyed by antibiotics, the body can no longer remove the tumor, or added tissue, so it is encapsulated and remains in place.

The Missing Lung Cancer Study

The biological program of the lungs was inadvertently revealed by an interesting series of experiments on field mice and hamsters. To prove that smoking caused cancer, medical researchers locked field mice in smoke-filled chambers. In time, they determined that all the field mice developed lung cancers. Under the same experiment, none of the hamsters developed lung cancer.

Why?

When you understand the evolutionary differences between field mice and hamsters, this seeming contradiction is not difficult to explain. Field mice live above ground and hamsters live below. Between natural wildfires and farmers burning their fields before planting or after harvest, field mice have evolved to associate smoke with danger. Therefore, if field mice are trapped in a smoke-filled chamber, their fear of death triggers the lung cancer biological program. Since hamsters live underground and are not directly threatened by fires raging above them, they do not have this fear-of-death biological program.

So where is this original study? Buried.

Unfortunately, conventional science tends to support whoever is funding it. After these experiments were conducted, the only results published were those that related to field mice. *Not to hamsters.* Obviously, the latter did not support the desired conclusion: Smoking causes lung cancer.

Metastasis Hypothesis

We have been conditioned to believe by conventional medicine that metastasized cancer occurs when cancer cells break from tumors and swim through your bloodstream or lymphatic system and attack other organs. Let us examine this statement through a different lens.

The most common secondary or metastatic cancers are of the lung, liver, and lymph glands. Isn't it strange that in paired organs like breasts and testicles, cancer generally only affects one organ and does not metastasize to the second organ when it is made from the same tissue and lives right next door?

According to an NIH (National Institutes of Health) study published in 2019, *National Trends of Bilateral Breast Cancer Incidence in the United States,* the incidence of bilateral breast cancer (cancer in both breasts) increased significantly from 1.4% in 1975 to 2.9% in 2014. Even though the incidence has more than doubled since 1975, in more than 97% of breast cancer cases, cancer does not metastasize to the second breast.[4]

In a testicular cancer research study published by NIH in 2017, *Synchronous bilateral testis cancer: clinical and oncological management,* Synchronous Bilateral Testis Cancer is a rare event. It represents only 0.5–1% of all new cases of testicular cancer. In 99% of testicular cancer cases, the cancer does not metastasize to the second testicle.[5]

The Lymphatic System

In the Germanic Healing Knowledge system, the lymphatic system is affected by a self-esteem conflict that results in the inability to clean or remove an internal burden, e.g., swelling and inflammation of an organ. The lymphatic system closest to that organ is affected. Most commonly, it is the lymph nodes under the armpit next to the affected breast, or in the groin for testicular cancer.

Is it possible that when you have a painful swelling on your breast or testicle, you suffer from a self-esteem conflict of being unable to rid yourself of something unpleasant?

The lymph nodes reduce in size during the first, conflict active phase, and swell up, become painful, and are replenished during the second, healing or repair phase. You only become aware of the problem in the lymph glands once you have resolved the self-esteem conflict of having a painful swelling on your breast or testicle. This is typically either after the organ has healed or been removed via surgery.

It is at this point that medical doctors tell you the cancer has spread to your lymph nodes, a terrifying prognosis for any patient. The swelling of the lymph gland next to the affected organ is merely a part of the healing process of the lymph gland. The lymph gland experiences ulceration, or tissue loss, during the conflict of having a painful swelling on the organ. Once the conflict has been resolved, i.e., the pain in the organ has gone, the lymph glands start to heal. This involves pain and inflammation, the same way the body heals when you cut your finger.

At the end of the healing phase, the lymph glands have a greater capacity than before the conflict. This is the body's way of protecting against future possible conflicts of the same kind. The purpose of these biological programs is to make you stronger.

Given this information, we need to seriously reconsider what is causing metastatic cancers. Are medical diagnoses and treatment protocols responsible for triggering new biological conflict shocks that cause secondary cancers? These are questions worth thinking about.

CHAPTER 5
WHY A TERMINAL CANCER DIAGNOSIS IS INCORRECT

*I*n Dr. Hamer's medical science, the Germanic Healing Knowledge, there is no such diagnosis as terminal cancer.

Just because a medical doctor has given you a terminal diagnosis, it does not mean it is the end of the road. A large hospital can give you the best organ-level diagnosis of your symptoms. Unfortunately, the doctors working there are only allowed to manage those symptoms with drugs, surgery, and radiation.

Treating organ-level symptoms is never going to solve your health challenge. You must connect the dots from the organ, through the brain, to the unexpected distress that affected your psyche and resolve the conflict in your life that triggered this chain of events.

The Brain's Role in Disease

Dr. Hamer made the essential connection between the psyche, the brain, and our body's organs. He determined biological programs, or diseases, as the doctors call them, are caused by our psyche's perception of unexpected, distressing, external events (except for poisoning, injuries from accidents and nutritional deficiency diseases, e.g., scurvy through a lack of vitamin C).

From my years as a consultant, I know that when we want to solve business problems, we must look at input-process-output. In health terms: The input is the life experience that causes the unexpected biological conflict shock/trauma. *Processing happens in the brain.* The outputs are the biological changes which affect organ performance levels.

A good example to demonstrate this is what medical science calls phantom limb pain, when amputees still experience pain in a limb after amputation. The Cleveland Clinic reports that eight out of ten people who have limbs amputated still experience pain in the limb despite its absence.[1] This begs the question: How does someone feel pain in a limb that is no longer there? The answer: The pain is in the brain, not the limb/organ. It does not matter whether the organ is still there or not. The biological program, which is resulting in pain, is still running in the brain.

The brain is the control center where the program runs, and the organ expresses the program. You can never solve the problem at the organ level. The organ expresses the symptoms of the program; it is not the "CAUSE."

Having an organ removed has little or no effect on the risk of getting cancer. If you want to eliminate your risk of cancer by removing organs, it appears the only viable option would be to cut off your head. And this is far from an ideal solution.

My Work with Cancer Patients

Over the years, I have helped hundreds of cancer patients, many who had already been given a terminal diagnosis. More than half of the people I helped not only received an incorrect terminal diagnosis, but their primary medical diagnosis was also incorrect. Some of these situations were true horror stories.

If you learn to read brain CT scans like Dr. Hamer, you can see someone's entire health history recorded in the tissues of their brain.

To recap, when we experience an unexpected biological conflict shock, it triggers a chain of events that impacts the psyche, brain, and organ in an instant — like an electric shock. This unexpected distress leaves a physical impression, a set of "target rings" on the relay in the brain that is associated with a specific organ, and it also starts a physiological process — an adaptation — in the organ itself. These foci can be seen in the brain via a computed tomography (CT) scan.

Lung Cancer

A man in his 70s was sent home to die of terminal, stage IV lung cancer. He came to see me with his son, as he had lost his voice and could not speak. When I reviewed his medical records, I saw he had been diagnosed with biopsy-proven lung cancer of the alveoli. The conflict associated with this, according to Dr. Hamer, would have been a death-fright conflict. I asked him to get a brain CT done. When I checked it, there was nothing to be seen on the brain relay of the lung alveoli. *Zero activity.*

I checked the bronchi (the air tubes in the lungs) relay on his brain CT scan. The medical diagnosis was wrong, even though it was "biopsy proven." His problem was with his bronchi, not the alveoli. The bronchi are affected by what Dr. Hamer described as a "territorial fear conflict."

Throughout human history, a challenge to our territory meant a fight to the death. During a territorial challenge, the bronchi widen to get more oxygen to our muscles. In this way, we have more strength and endurance to outlast whomever or whatever is posing a challenge to our territory.

After a few counseling sessions, this man's son explained that his father lives in their home. His grandson is his pride and joy.

One day, his daughter-in-law came home from work in a bad mood. Annoyed by her son, she slapped him on the head and sent him to his room. The grandfather was mortified and felt the punishment was unjust. He lost his voice because he could not speak about the problem.

Once we understood the cause of his ill health, the family met. His daughter-in-law apologized to her son and father-in-law. She admitted she was wrong, and it would never happen again. Thus, the problem was resolved. In a few weeks, the grandfather's voice returned, and his lungs healed. He was back in full health.

I found the next case very suspicious: A man explained to me that he went to the hospital for problems with his wrist. The doctor instructed the man to get a chest X-ray. He tried to explain to the doctor that the problem was in his wrist and not his chest. The doctor insisted he get a chest X-ray, and then kept him waiting for hours to get the results.

He was told, "You might have lung cancer; please come back in two months and we will do another X-ray." After two months of worrying about the possibility of dying from lung cancer, the patient went back to the doctor and had another chest X-ray. He was diagnosed with lung cancer. As explained, Dr. Hamer believed that lung cancer of the alveoli is caused by a death-fright conflict. I always wonder whether that doctor had studied Dr. Hamer's work and then used that knowledge to generate new business.

Liver Cancer

A liver cancer patient consulted me after receiving an aggressive, ductal liver cancer diagnosis. He had just had his gallbladder and 50% of his liver removed. I asked him to get a brain CT scan done. According to Dr. Hamer, unlike liver parenchyma cancer which responds to a starvation conflict, ductal liver cancer is caused by "territorial anger."

When I looked at his brain relay for the liver ducts, it was unremarkable. The surgery had been completely unnecessary. For comparison, I showed the patient my own brain CT scan. It had *much* more activity regarding territorial anger on the liver ducts' relay. This man had his gallbladder and half of his liver removed for absolutely no reason.

After the surgery, the hospital tried to make even more money by inviting him to take part in a clinical trial — in the event the problem returned. According to his oncologist, a relapse was highly probable. When he asked for details on the clinical trial, his doctors seemed indignant that he even questioned it, and information was reluctantly provided. After reading the small print, he discovered that the drugs used in the clinical trial had a 25% chance of causing kidney failure. Horrified, he declined. This man described his whole hospital experience as a trip to the gates of hell and back again.

Brain Cancer

According to Dr. Hamer, there is no such thing as brain cancer. Neurons in the brain do not multiply after birth. The only cells in the brain that multiply are called glial cells. Diagnosed by medical doctors as glioblastoma or brain cancer, these glial cells are harmless and have a biological purpose. Glial cells are reconnective tissue that repair the brain and are simply finishing the healing phase from a conflict shock lesion (Hamer foci). Dr. Hamer's music therapy aids in the healing of these situations very well. You can read more about this in chapter 8.

Dr. Hamer reported that medical doctors cannot read brain CT scans.[2] Each time somebody came to me with a brain cancer diagnosis, I put Dr. Hamer's assertion to the test. I had these patients take their brain CT scans to five different neurologists and instructed them NOT to disclose their previous brain cancer diagnosis.

Every time, without exception, the neurologist said nothing was wrong, and they should take a pain killer.

Next, I sent them to five more neurologists. This time, when they showed those very same brain CT scans, they disclosed their previous brain cancer diagnosis. On every occasion, the neurologists confirmed their brain cancer diagnosis. The patient was now convinced that their medical doctors had no idea what they were doing, and they had been misdiagnosed. This opened the door for me to help them with a correct diagnosis of their brain (health) problem.

No Cancer

In another instance, a woman in her 60s had received seventeen rounds of chemotherapy until she ran out of money. Told by her doctors that nothing else could be done, she was sent home to die. When I went through her medical records, I discovered that a blood test was the only diagnostic procedure upon which her doctors had based their therapy decision. During her annual health check, the doctors found cancer markers in her blood. She was told to start chemo immediately.

I had her get a CT scan of her brain. In this woman's case, there was absolutely nothing wrong with her. She was not terminally ill, she did not have cancer, and never should have had chemotherapy. Fortunately, she took this as great news and went back to living her life. She moved on, accepting the whole episode as a bad life experience.

My years of experience in dealing with these types of reprehensible misdiagnosis stories have left me incredibly skeptical of both the capability and competence of the modern medical system.

Inka Sattler, A Beacon of Hope

I recommend reading the autobiography of one of Dr. Hamer's patients, Inka Sattler. Before experiencing her own health challenges, Inka was a nurse in a cancer ward. One of her duties was to administer chemotherapy. After years of witnessing how this destroyed patients' health, she swore that if she ever got cancer, she would never let herself be admitted to a hospital and receive chemotherapy.

True to her word, Inka survived seven cancer diagnoses, including bone cancer which led to paraplegia and left her confined to a bed for months. Finally, she was given a terminal diagnosis and sent to a hospice. Refusing to give up and die, Inka walked out of the hospice alive. Decades after she was given a death sentence by her doctors, Inka did finally leave us in 2021. Her story remains as an extraordinary testament and an inspiring read.[3] Imagine: Inka was a nurse in a cancer ward and had to unlearn everything she had been taught before she was able to beat her terminal diagnosis.

CHAPTER 6
SWITCH OFF TERMINAL CANCER PAIN

*A*ny palliative care professional can give you a detailed description of the excruciating, full-body pain often experienced by patients who have been diagnosed with a "terminal, incurable cancer." In the face of impending death, this pain is usually treated with powerful painkillers, e.g., morphine and fentanyl.

However, if we understand the root cause and the biological purpose of the program that caused it, we can switch off the pain. Let me explain how pain related to a terminal diagnosis works. We have a membrane enveloping our bones called the periosteum. The periosteum contains all the bone's nerves and is extremely sensitive. The excruciating pain from a broken bone is caused by the torn or damaged layer of periosteum.

I have experienced periosteum pain and describe it as "twenty-on-ten. "Think of the worst pain you have ever experienced. On a scale of one to ten, I would call that pain a 10 (ten-on-ten pain). Periosteum pain is double that (twenty-on-ten pain). People who have never experienced this off-the-chart pain can consider themselves lucky. This is when the doctors start administering morphine and fentanyl.

What is deeply saddening, and what doctors do not realize, is that their diagnosis of terminal cancer and impending death, triggers the start of the patient's periosteum pain.

Fear of Brutal Separation

Dr. Hamer determined that the biological conflict causing periosteum pain is a fear-of-brutal-separation conflict. Periosteum pain is nature's danger warning alarm. This means that you (your psyche) are afraid of being separated from your body (dying). The way the periosteum pain program works is as follows: After years of different treatments, a doctor says, "I have some unwelcome news. There is nothing more that we can do to help you. You have X amount of time left to live. Go home and get your affairs in order."

If you believe the doctor's diagnosis, and you are not ready to die, this will trigger your periosteum. Soon after receiving this fatal diagnosis, you will begin experiencing excruciating, twenty-on-ten, full-body pain. It is when the pain finally becomes unbearable that doctors administer morphine and other end-of-life drugs. Still, as unbelievable as it sounds, it is possible to switch off that unbearable pain like a light switch.

Refusing to accept being sent home to die and instead saying, "I disagree with your diagnosis," empowers the mind and body. You will not develop this full-body pain since the fear of being separated from your material body has not been triggered.

The biological program of periosteum pain in Germanic Healing Knowledge is called Rheumatoid Arthritis in Conventional Medicine.

Turning Off the Pain

Dr. Hamer discovered there are two ways to switch off what doctors call disease, or what he called biological programs. The first is to find a biological solution to the problem in real life, which is not applicable in this case: *Before* you heard the diagnosis, you would have needed the knowledge and wisdom that no diagnosis is a death sentence. If this had been the case, the periosteum pain would not have been triggered.

The second way to switch off the biological program is to consciously connect the original conflict shock that began the biological program with the symptoms it triggered. This conscious awareness can switch off the symptoms. In this case, the doctor's terminal diagnosis triggered your periosteum pain, but more importantly, *it was your belief in the doctor's diagnosis.*

Try this exercise to switch off the pain: First, visualize the discussion where the doctor delivered the devastating news that you are going to die. Next, consciously connect that discussion with your full-body pain. Have a conversation with your psyche along these lines:

"I am visualizing the discussion with my doctor, where he/she told me that there are no more treatments available, and that I have 3–6 months to live. That diagnosis triggered a fear of dying before I was ready to go. Consequently, my fear caused the periosteum layer of skin over my bones to sound my body's ultimate red alert, this twenty-on-ten pain. **I am not going to die; my doctor's diagnosis is incorrect. They are only treating the symptoms and not the cause of the problem. Please switch off the pain.**"

Tell this to yourself even if you do not believe it for now. What happened to the twenty-on-ten pain? It is possible that you first downgraded the pain from twenty-on-ten to four or five-on-ten instead of switching it off completely. Still, this is also a good outcome. Pain that is four-on-ten is manageable.

This technique has saved me from many difficult situations, including periosteum pain affecting my spine and arm. There is just one catch: If you switch off biological programs involving pain without fixing the real-life problems that are causing them, these programs can easily be switched back on again. They came for a reason and will persist until we resolve them in real life.

If you still believe, somewhere in the back of your mind, that your disease is really going to kill you, as soon as there is a reminder or trigger that takes you back to your doctor's terminal diagnosis, the pain switches on again. The pain will only go away for good when you find a real-life, practical solution to your problem(s). In this situation, fortunately, all that is necessary is acquiring knowledge (a process you are starting by reading this book).

More importantly, you must genuinely believe it.

Discovering the Triggers

The next element important to understand is how these triggers work. Triggers, or stimuli that remind us of an unresolved conflict shock, are what lead to chronic illnesses. A disease becomes chronic when any given biological program that is responsible for certain symptoms is activated repeatedly. This happens due to the presence of one or more triggers.

Imagine the following example: You are walking down a dark city street at night when suddenly someone jumps out from behind a parked truck, bashes you over the head, and steals your money. In the split second you are being attacked, your psyche, or subconscious, takes a snapshot and records all the sensory details of the situation. This often includes sounds, smells, noises, and even food, if you were eating at the time of the attack.

After that traumatic event, any time you find yourself in a similar situation, i.e., on a dark street lined with cars, your psyche triggers your fight-or-flight response. If the person who mugged you jumped out from behind a black pickup truck, your psyche can record this type and color of vehicle as one of the key factors for indicating imminent danger. Every time you see a black pickup truck, your psyche will put you into fight-or-flight mode. The body responds with a racing heart, flushed or pale skin, dilated pupils, dry mouth, and sweaty hands.[1] Your psyche is screaming "Danger! Danger!" so you do not get hurt again.

Unfortunately, a real problem associated with this evolutionary warning system is that it reaches far beyond the surface. If you do not consciously remember that your attacker jumped out from behind a black pickup truck, you will now have an "irrational" fear of these vehicles. Similarly, for example, if you were eating an apple at the time of the attack, the next time you eat an apple, it could trigger fight-or-flight anxiety, or even an allergic reaction. This all makes perfect sense when you understand how it works. If you consciously connect these triggers to the night you were attacked, you can switch them off.

The following is an example from my own life:

While riding down the highway on a scooter with my girlfriend in Bali, Indonesia, a crack about four inches wide and twenty feet long suddenly opened in the road. With no time to react, the front wheel plunged into the crack. My girlfriend and I flew over the handlebars and suffered injuries. Fifteen years later, I bought a bike to get around town. Whenever I saw a seam in the road where two pieces of cement slabs or tarmac met, my heart started racing and my mouth went dry; I had all the symptoms of acute anxiety. It took me a good while to work out why this was happening. At the time, though, I had only just started studying Dr. Hamer's medical discoveries and had little experience in connecting the dots.

After six months of suffering inexplicable anxiety attacks while bike-riding, I finally remembered the 1997 incident in Bali. When I consciously connected the past accident with the present anxiety, I stopped suffering the attacks. Just like that, I switched off the trigger. It still blows my mind every time I flip off one of those switches.

Fortunately, the psyche does not always react to every sign of danger. It only puts you in fight-or-flight mode when encountering a unique stimulus involved in an unresolved biological conflict shock. With the aim of increasing your chances of survival, it reminds you of previously experienced danger in connection with this stimulus and turns the biological program back on again.

The psyche is in charge when the conscious mind is acting on autopilot (which is actually most of the time). This is especially true when we are overwhelmed and cannot pay attention to everything. When you inform your conscious mind of what your psyche is trying to do, your psyche steps back and disarms the triggers that cause anxiety and panic attacks. Once you consciously connect the biological stimulus from a past traumatic event, your psyche says, "Okay, you have finally made the connection in your conscious awareness. Now that you have come to terms with it, I do not need to keep reminding you." Your psyche will either immediately delete the program for good, or at least it will not turn it back on again.

Healing Death-Sentence Triggers

When a doctor surprises you with a death sentence, the situation will create triggers and reminders of this terrifying moment. All the sensory input from that moment can act as a trigger: sights, sounds, smells, textures, foods, etc. They work in the same way as if you had been ambushed in the dark.

For example, if you were in a hospital setting, details such as a long white coat, the smell of disinfectants, or even the music you heard in the waiting area, could trigger the pain to start up again. If your partner were there, they could inadvertently become a trigger too, or even the specific outfit they wore that day.

Please note that if you use the technique of consciously connecting the doctor's death sentence to the periosteum pain and successfully switch it off, and the pain starts up again in the next few days, this means you have been reminded or triggered by a memory of that trauma. If that happens, build a clear picture of everything related to that traumatic moment in time. When you find the trigger, say to yourself, for example:

"I remember the song that was playing in the doctor's office when he/she delivered the death sentence, and I just heard that song again. I know it is a reminder or trigger of that traumatic experience. I am not going to die; please switch off the pain."

If you have correctly identified the trigger, it will switch the pain back off again. There are often multiple tracks, or reminders, that can switch the pain back on again, so you will need to work to identify them all. Once you have switched them off, the pain will not return, unless your fear-of-death conflict relapses. Ideally, by this time, you will have reviewed Dr. Hamer's Scientific Chart and learned about the biological conflict shock (root cause) behind your health challenge and have made some progress toward solving the problem in your everyday life.

This technique triggers a process of cathartic healing that is almost impossible to believe, until you experience it for yourself. I would like to repeat what I strongly advise to those who come to me for help: Do not believe anything I recommend until you have personal experience with switching off biological programs. Never convince yourself of anything until personally verifying it for yourself. Once you go through this exercise and are successful in either downgrading or switching off the pain altogether, you will believe in its validity.

By now, you may have guessed why I prefer to work with those who have been given a terminal diagnosis. Generally, but with rare exceptions, people are either unprepared or unable to listen to any alternative advice — aside from which plant or supplement is the best for solving their problems — until a pill is no longer an option. This is especially the case when their recovery involves taking responsibility for their own health, or the lack thereof.

In my experience, people sent home to die by conventional medical doctors often become incredibly open-minded. At that point, they are prepared to listen and learn how their body functions. It comes back to the old saying, "When people are ready to change, they change. They never do it before then, and sometimes they die before they get around to it."

Life is full of choices. Only when you understand the root cause of your health challenges and make the necessary changes in your life to reverse the biological chain of events and the triggers that make them reoccur, will you fully recover your health.

CHAPTER 7
THE REALITIES OF CANCER RESEARCH

*I*n my years of studying cancer and the cancer industry, my experience has been that if a cancer research report does not support maintenance of the status quo, it is buried, and buried deep. This applies equally to reports that show the results of current practices in a negative light, as well as those that demonstrate significant breakthroughs outside of chemotherapy, radiation, or surgery.

Cancer research is a dangerous occupation. It is common for doctors and researchers to be buried along with their reports. There are websites dedicated to tracking the unexplainable deaths of people in the cancer research industry, as well as doctors who use alternative medical practices.[1] Dr. Hamer experienced this personally and survived many attempts on his life.

Below I detail some concealed cancer research reports.

1993 Neustadt Austria - 90% Survival Rate

As mentioned earlier, in 1993 Dr. Hamer was prosecuted for practicing medicine without a license. The Public Prosecutor's Office of Neustadt subpoenaed 6,500 of Dr. Hamer's patients' files and called them all to find out their current state of health. Many had been declared terminally ill before being referred to Dr. Hamer. The prosecutor had to admit in court that over 6,000 were not only alive, but in full health. **That is a recovery rate of over 90%.** Dr. Hamer was subsequently given a six-month suspended prison sentence.[2]

1997 Cologne Germany - 85% Survival Rate

Dr. Hamer was prosecuted again in 1997 in Cologne Germany for practicing medicine without a license. He was given a nineteen-month prison sentence and served twelve months. As part of Dr. Hamer's defense, Marc Fréchet, a psychologist who specialized in cancer patients, was called to testify in the case.

Marc Fréchet spent years studying and using Dr. Hamer's medical research findings and had an 85% survival rate with his patients who refused conventional medical treatments.

Below is a transcript of his testimony published on August 20, 1997 by Helmut Pilhar, Dr. Hamer's appointed successor.[3]

Marc Fréchet to the Court in Cologne - Testimony

Marc Fréchet, Clinical Psychologist - Medical and Psychological Oncology

Testimonial

Your Honours,

I am aware that this statement may be used in this court. I am aware of and accept the possible consequences of the following statement with regard to your jurisdiction.

I have been practicing as a freelance clinical psychologist since 1978. For nine years I practiced in the field of medical oncology at the Paul Brousse Clinic in Villejuif, in direct collaboration with Prof. G. Mathe. Funding was provided by the Association Claude Bernard.

My activities were as follows: Every Thursday I was busy with consultations all day. Individuals who consulted me were burdened with somatic symptoms that presented themselves as blood disorders or tumors. All these patients were referred to me by the attending physicians at the clinic.

During these nine years, I have had consultations with about 1,000 people. Among these patients were both adults and children. Outside of consultation hours, I was involved in my area of practice, research. This research consisted in reviewing statements of numerous people, regarding the psychological aspect of cancer suffering. The reason for conducting this review was the following:

Faced with my patients' despair or depression and search for a miraculous and immediate treatment, I attempted to find an inner meaning to the illness instead of seeking solutions from the outside. I guided them to identify their daily problems as related to their suffering, to approach the situation from a different angle. Since my area of knowledge is not in medicine, patients were encouraged to tell me about their symptoms, complaints, and the consequences they experienced, both positive and negative.

After recording the various hammers of fate encountered by these persons, we identified certain general causes. If these results had been intended for publication, it would have been concluded that all individuals who experienced such psychological problems were most likely to have suffered organic damage eventually in their lives.

Our permanent search in the course of this work was to identify as precisely as possible the emotional sensation in connection with the organ symptoms. Here is an example: In connection with Breast Cancer,[4] five problem areas were identified.

In my opinion, Dr. Hamer lists as many varieties as we also found. Medically, I worked out the biological identification of breast cancer through my work in Villejuif. Dr. Hamer's method has allowed me to more specifically determine the emotional disturbances associated with this somatic symptomatology. When the available old studies of women and men are analyzed, the distinct types of cancer can be classified according to the categories defined by Dr. Hamer.

We can — independently of Dr. Hamer's work — using the data on the patients we examined in detail, confirm the method developed by Dr. Hamer one hundred percent.

Our concern was to identify the patients' feelings about their disease as accurately and completely as possible. If I were to present the results of our psychosomatic analysis of the problems expressed by our patients to Dr. Hamer, he would be able to precisely assign the pathology of the patients to the psychological problem areas.

As a former general practitioner at the hospital, I cared for 3 distinct groups of patients:

- Group A. consisting of 380 individuals (41%) who received medical treatment
- Group B. consisting of 215 individuals (26%) who decisively refused medical treatment and
- Group C. consisting of 312 individuals (33%) who appeared for consultation only once.

Regardless of which medical treatment the patients followed or not, I can only confirm that an intimate understanding of the biological and psychological mechanisms associated with the medical symptoms always led to an improvement in the patient's situation. Many of them are still doing well today. Their lives have improved in quality and inner peace.

Looking back over the six years of research in Villejuif, 285 of 604 individuals survived as of June 29, 1994, i.e., 47%.

Of those survivors:

- 102 i.e., 28% belonged to Group A and
- 183 i.e., 85% belonged to Group B.

I cared for the patients in Group A according to their wishes, averaging 8 hours per person. Group B patients were entitled to a minimum of 40 hours per person. Both groups had the opportunity to contact us outside of the consultations, by phone.

In summary, I would like to state that most of the deceased patients died from their anxiety, due to biological fatigue and their emotional isolation, from the same causes that led to their illness.

With these short remarks I hope to have given you, Your Honours, a small insight into the richness that the occupation with the findings and results of Dr. Hamer brings with it. I wished I could have worked alongside him.

Even though Marc Fréchet presented compelling evidence to the court that Dr. Hamer's approach to helping cancer patients delivered significantly improved outcomes in terms of survival rates, Dr. Hamer was sent to prison.

Like many other brave cancer research specialists who had a story that mainstream medicine did not want told, Marc Fréchet was buried, along with his cancer research report. The blogpost titled "Marc Fréchet — Obituary by Dr. Hamer" was published on Helmut Pilhar's website on January 15, 1998.[5]

Marc Fréchet - Obituary by Dr. Hamer

Marc Fréchet had been asked by his boss Prof. Mathe, one of the three bosses besides Prof. Israel and Prof. Schwarzenberg, from the well-known national cancer treatment center Villejuif near Paris, to find out how many patients die if "nothing is done."

He was allowed to provide psychotherapy to both groups, the chemo-treated patients and the untreated. But of course, the untreated patients, mostly untreatable, i.e., incurable cases, had also already suffered the diagnosis and prognosis shock. Usually, such patients die at the same percentage rate as the chemo-treated ones.

It was not planned that Marc Fréchet would be explaining Germanic New Medicine to them. When it finally became known what he had been doing, and that over 85% of the untreated, who had found their way out of the panic through Germanic New Medicine, survived, and even 28% of the chemo-treated patients, who had also found their way out of the panic through Germanic New Medicine, survived, he was immediately thrown out of the hospital.

The tragedy: Fréchet now wanted to publish his findings but had suffered a self-worth conflict "I can't do this" when being sacked, with osteolysis in the femoral neck at the organ level.

A few days before finishing his documentation "Now I've done it," his osteolysis went into the healing phase and his groin swelled up.

Although aware of Germanic New Medicine, he rashly went to a hospital near Paris to be examined. Something very strange happened there. Fréchet was given morphine, possibly under a pretext, possibly also without his knowledge, after which he did not wake up.

After 10 days, Marc Fréchet was dead.

Particularly macabre: His boss, Prof. Mathe, had himself been treated by me and my friends more than 10 years ago for a bronchial carcinoma in line with Germanic New Medicine — without chemo. Since recovering, he resumed using chemo in patients — well aware of the 98% pseudo therapy mortality.

Marc Fréchet died as a martyr for the Germanic New Medicine.

Dr. Ryke Geerd Hamer

2004 Chemotherapy Oncology Study - 2% Survival Rate

In 2004, a group of oncologists in the Northern Sydney Cancer Centre in Australia carried out a clinical oncology study. They assessed the five-year survival rate of cancer patients who only had chemotherapy as a treatment, i.e., no surgery or radiation. They analyzed 72,903 patients with twenty types of cancer. Only 1,690 were still alive after five years, a five-year survival rate of 2.3%.[6]

The oncologists believed there must be a problem with Australia's medical treatment system, so they replicated the study in America. They doubled the sample size and analyzed the cases of 154,971 cancer patients. Again, these patients only had chemotherapy as a treatment, no surgery or radiation. After five years, 3,306 were still alive, a survival rate of 2.1%.

Let that sink in.

The oncologists carrying out the study concluded:

"In an environment of scarce resources and cost-containment, there is a need for evidence-based assessment before any new or previously accepted treatment is accepted as standard practice. To justify the continued funding and availability of drugs used in cytotoxic chemotherapy,

a rigorous evaluation of the cost-effectiveness and impact on quality of life is urgently required."

The oncologists' study was subsequently buried.

Conventional medicine has a standard that if a treatment protocol does not help at least 30% of the people who take the treatment, it should be discontinued. Why then do they still use chemotherapy as a treatment when, according to oncologists in Australia, it kills more than 97% of the people who take it?

The existing medical system, that has five-year survival rates in single digits, is protected by the medical and legal systems. According to PubMed, medical treatments are the third leading cause of death in the US.[7] Johns Hopkins reports that 10% of deaths in the US each year are caused by medical errors.[8] Doctors who attempt to practice principles of new medical discoveries that have demonstrated success rates in the 80% and 90% range (which include many people who had already been sent home to die by conventional medicine) are thrown in prison and, in some cases, murdered.

In my opinion, it all comes down to money. Conventional medicine is a multi-trillion-dollar business. A doctor's favorite prescription is pharmaceutical drugs for life. If Dr. Hamer's medical discoveries become mainstream, conventional medicine is out of business. There is no price too high to ensure that this does not happen.

CHAPTER 8
HEALING WITH MUSIC THERAPY

*L*ater in his career, Dr. Hamer spent years exploring the healing power of music. Once again, he made even more extraordinary discoveries.

Working closely with an Italian music professor and classical pianist, Prof. Giovanna Conti, they made what Dr. Hamer described as the "greatest therapeutic discovery in the history of mankind."

When you listen to music with a melody that has been composed according to the principles of the Golden Ratio and Fibonacci Sequence played at 432 hertz (Hz), it will help you remove oedema from your brain and return to homeostasis (the natural, healthy, rhythmic state of nervous system function) by restoring your normal psyche-brain-organ harmony. If you are in the first of the two phases, the conflict-active phase, the vibrational frequency can downgrade your conflict. After you resolve your conflict and enter the repair phase, it can fast-track the healing process.

Biphasic Music Pattern

In 2007, while Prof. Giovanna Conti was deepening her understanding of Germanic Healing Knowledge, she discovered that certain types of Western classical music followed the same pattern as Dr. Hamer's 2nd Biological Law, The Law of Two Phases. After analyzing this in depth, she shared her work with Dr. Hamer.

Impressed, Dr. Hamer asked Prof. Conti to analyze his song, *Mein Studentenmädchen* (My Student Maiden). In 1976, Dr. Hamer had composed this song for his beloved first wife and mother of his children, Sigrid Oldenburg, for their 20th wedding anniversary. Prof. Conti determined that the structure of *Mein Studentenmädchen* also corresponded exactly with the pattern of Dr. Hamer's 2nd Biological Law and chose the song as the prototype for her subsequent research.

She went on to discover that many classical masterpieces, including ones by Mozart, Beethoven, Chopin, and Schubert, also followed, in detail, the same pattern that Dr. Hamer recognized in the 2nd Biological Law of the Germanic Healing Knowledge. Furthermore, Prof. Conti found that the biphasic pattern she observed in those masterpieces, and in *Mein Studentenmädchen,* also corresponded with the proportions of the Golden Section, or Golden Ratio. In a nutshell, this is the mathematical principle that can be found everywhere in nature and is expressed by the Fibonacci Sequence. This principle is understood to have a geometric expression that is referred to as "godlike in its natural perfection."[1]

432 Hertz Frequency Music

In the 19th century, classical music was tuned at A=432 Hz, a frequency that is also mathematically consistent with the Fibonacci Sequence (also called Verdi tuning). In the early 20th century, however, the Rockefeller Foundation researched music frequencies. They discovered that if you increase the tuning frequency of music from 432 Hz to 440 Hz, among other dubious effects, worker bees work harder and faster. In 1939, and again in 1953, international conferences organized in London by the British Standards Institute started a process of the adoption of A=440 Hz, as promoted by the Rockefeller Foundation. In time, this became the universal standard for tuning musical instruments.[2]

Healing with Music

Dr. Hamer focused on the application of *Mein Studentenmädchen*. While playing the song at 432 Hz during the treatment of certain diseases, he discovered that *Mein Studentenmädchen* put disease programs on hold. He said the 432 Hz version of the song, with his vocals accompanied by a cello, was twice as effective as the 440 Hz version performed by a professional orchestra. If you listen to Dr. Hamer's song 24/7 (this can be played at a barely audible level in the background), it puts the disease process into stasis, similar to how a woman's body goes into stasis during the second and third trimester of pregnancy.

The extraordinary healing properties of *Mein Studentenmädchen* was "accidentally" discovered by a seven-year-old Austrian girl. For months, she had suffered from chronic bronchitis. Distraught over his daughter's illness, her father purchased Dr. Hamer's book, *Die Archaischen Melodien* (The Archaic Melody), which included a DVD of the song. Intuitively, this young girl was infatuated with *Mein Studentenmädchen* and listened to it day and night. Three days later, to the astonishment of her parents, she walked out of her bedroom in full health.

In time, Dr. Hamer observed extraordinary results in the people who listened to his music. This was especially the case for people suffering from conflict constellations (two active conflicts on directly opposite sides of the brain that trigger major behavior changes), like children with Down Syndrome and autism, and even major health challenges like cancer. He found that it was beneficial for reducing, or in many cases, completely eliminating symptoms.

I gave the music to my friend whose four-year-old son, at the time, was highly autistic. While his son slept, my friend had the music quietly playing in the background. Within a year, the boy had transformed from a quiet and despondent, developmentally challenged four-year-old who could barely communicate, to a highly engaging, outgoing, fun-loving, five-year-old.

Another example is the previously mentioned man who had come to me with 50% of his liver removed. He reported that when he listened to Dr. Hamer's music, his pain subsided to the point where he did not need to use any medications. As soon as he switched off the music, his pain levels would start to increase dramatically.

If you would like to watch Dr. Hamer explain the magic of his music therapy, visit his publishing company's web page for "Video Presentation on Mein Studentenmädchen."[3] You can purchase Dr. Hamer's healing music or his books on music therapy through his website.[4] Prof. Conti's book, The Biological Meaning of Music, is also included. Use Dr. Hamer's music therapy to put your disease progression on hold. This will buy you some time to find a GNM/GHk consultant to help you start resolving the biological conflicts responsible for your health issues.

CHAPTER 9
LEARN GHK/GNM TO HELP YOURSELF AND OTHERS

Dr. Hamer's Scientific Chart of Germanic New Medicine

*I*f you are interested in learning Dr. Hamer's medical discoveries, I strongly recommend buying a copy of his Scientific Chart of Germanic New Medicine. Aside from Dr. Hamer's publishing website and Helmut Pilhar's websites, where Dr. Hamer's original teachings are translated into English, the scientific chart and book are the only undiluted sources (or record) of his discoveries written in English. Otherwise, all his original publications are in German.[1]

Although the basics are relatively easy to grasp, learning the many intricacies of the medical science Dr. Hamer discovered reminds me of the old proverbial question, "How do you eat an elephant?" The answer, "One bite at a time."

GHk Pilhar Academy

There are no "certified" courses available yet because there is no certifying body for GHk anywhere on the planet. The best we can do is turn to the three experts Dr. Hamer appointed to the university he managed while he was alive. Of those three, only Helmut Pilhar was appointed as Dr. Hamer's official lecturer of what he called "the theory." This translates as the science of GHk.

For over two decades, Helmut taught GNM/GHk to countless audiences throughout the German-speaking world. In 2015, on his 80th birthday, Dr. Hamer directed Helmut to bring GHk to the masses via virtual learning. Helmut developed university-level certification courses in English with his appointed leaders, Nick Capetanis and Andi Locke Mears.[2] Shortly after completion, Helmut suddenly passed away.

These courses can be found through the GHk Pilhar Academy. Nick and Andi are continuing the academy with Dr. Hamer's and Helmut's material.[3] I studied under Ilsedora Laker, a long-time practitioner who worked closely with Dr. Hamer. I found her to be a great teacher of Germanic New Medicine/Germanic Healing Knowledge and highly recommend her classes.[4]

How Do I Contact a Consultant?

When you decide to set out on the journey back to health, I *strongly* recommend finding a consultant. As with any subject, you can acquire knowledge through research. I encourage every-one to learn as much as they can, but there is a huge difference between knowledge and wisdom. Dr. Hamer's medical discover-ies have many subtleties, and with an experienced consultant, you will have an invaluable partner on your healing journey. If there is not a consultant nearby, you can also achieve excellent results using video conferencing. I help people all over the world this way.

At the end of the day, you are responsible for your own health, or the lack thereof. In a counseling situation, your consultant can help guide you on your journey of self-healing, but your consul-tant cannot heal you — nor can a doctor.

There are rare cases you read about where extraordinary healers have healed people using energy or their hands. I am not one of those people. Personally, I have experienced that type of healing, and it truly is magical. However, for the other 99.9% of us, our only option is to heal ourselves. Fortunately, thanks to Dr. Hamer's medical discoveries, everyone can now learn to do so.

Finally, I urge you to visit my website Resources page for links to GHk practitioners around the world.[5]

CONCLUSION

I have been studying GNM/GHk for the last 10 years and, as Aristotle said, "The more you know, the more you know you don't know." The human body is a tremendously complex organism, and the challenges we face during our lives are virtually infinite in scope. Even though Dr. Hamer organized this new understanding of biology into a logical, scientific structure, learning GNM/GHk is a lifelong journey of discovery.

I can promise you that learning GNM/GHk comes with a huge return on your investment that pays out frequent dividends. It is truly life-changing. **Can you imagine your peace of mind when you have no more fear of disease? That is the place where I live.**

Come along and join me…

Fortunately, the hospitals will still be there if you ever need acute assistance on your road to recovery, like I did with my jaw. Furthermore, you will now be able to communicate with them from a position of knowledge (power), and not a state of confusion and helplessness.

This book is a brief introduction to some of the more important ideas contained in Dr. Hamer's work. I will follow up with a series of brief, organ and symptom-related books. Through my monthly digest called *The Healing Tribune — The Cause of Disease Made Simple,* I explore one disease and compare its cause(s) and cure from a Conventional Medicine and a Germanic Healing Knowledge perspective. Readers are left to decide which explanation is more compelling. There will be 500+ digests written over time, one for each disease.

If there is a specific health challenge you are facing and would like me to cover it, please email me with a brief description of your situation. I will prioritize health issues based on the greatest need.

With the knowledge contained in this book, you will be able to switch off the twenty-on-ten, full-body pain caused by a terminal diagnosis, like a light switch. If you listen to Dr. Hamer's healing music 24/7, you can put your disease process on hold and buy yourself some time to understand and address the real-life challenges that are causing your health issues. With patience and perseverance, you will be one of the thousands of people who have been lucky enough to discover Dr. Hamer's work. Like me, many of them have been able to resolve their health issues successfully.

Finally, if learning about Dr. Hamer's medical discoveries has been a eureka moment for you, as it was for me, I would be grateful if you could post a review of this book. As an independent author and publisher, even just one or two lines helps tremendously. Most importantly, please share your success stories about addressing health issues after learning GHk.

I wish you the best of luck on your healing journey.

Also by Danny Carroll

The Healing Tribune

The Cause Of Disease Made Simple

The CAUSE and SOLUTION for Breast Cancer Revealed

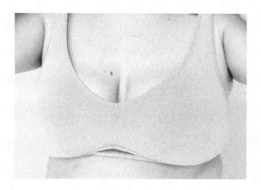

Breast Cancer Symptoms? Austrailian oncologists reported, women who take chemotherapy for breast cancer have a 5-year survival rate of 1.5%. Read this digest to discover a better way to solve the problem.

DANNY CARROLL

Short URL: **tht.fyi/bc**

The Healing Tribune

The Cause Of Disease Made Simple

The CAUSE and SOLUTION for Testicular Cancer Revealed

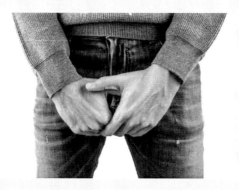

Testicular Cancer Symptoms? Australian oncologists reported, men who take chemotherapy for testicular cancer have a 5-year survival rate of 38–42%. Read this digest to learn a better way to solve the problem. I did.

DANNY CARROLL

Short URL: **tht.fyi/tc**

The Healing Tribune

The Cause Of Disease Made Simple

The CAUSE and SOLUTION for Atopic Dermatitis Revealed

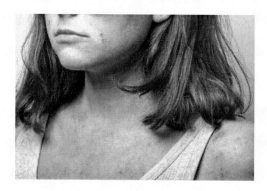

Atopic dermatits treatment. If you suffer from eczema, psoriasis, hives or urticaria, cold sores, herpes, rosacea and lupus erythematosus, chichenpox, measles, rubella, vitiligo, and warts, you will want to read this digest.

DANNY CARROLL

Short URL: **tht.fyi/ad**

The Healing Tribune

The Cause Of Disease Made Simple

The CAUSE and SOLUTION for IBS and Ulcerative Colitis Revealed

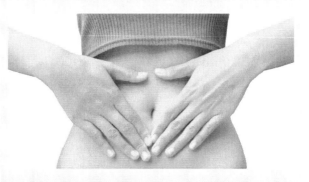

IBS symptoms? Learn to switch them off like a lights witch. I did. Identify the 'ugly' life problem that makes you angry. Practically solve that problem, and you will be free from the digestive stress that blights your life.

DANNY CARROLL

Short URL: **tht.fyi/ibs**

THE HEALING TRIBUNE

Sign up to claim a Free 400+ page e-book that includes the 'CAUSES' of nearly all known diseases, with over 500 case studies.

Plus, a FREE one-year course of 6–7-minute MP3 daily classes to start learning Germanic Healing Knowledge.

You'll also receive my free monthly installments of

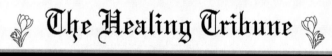

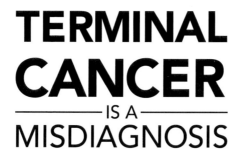

TERMINAL
CANCER
──── IS A ────
MISDIAGNOSIS

Discover A Palliative Care Alternative
Medicine You Can Survive

Edited by Anne Monet, Andrew Schlademan, & Laura Terry

ENDNOTES

I had initially included the long form URL in the footnotes but they were difficult to type out. I tried using publicly available short URLs, but many of the URLs were censored. Finally, I developed my own short URL, THT.FYI (The Healing Tribune For Your Information). Short URLs have been assigned to all footnotes starting with tht.fyi/. These are easy to type and no longer get censored.

Introduction

1. *The Costs of Cancer.* (n.d.). American Cancer Society Cancer Action Network. **tht.fyi/1million**

2. Dr. Hamer's Journey of Discovery

1. *The German/Germanic New Medicine.* (n.d.). The German New Medicine. **tht.fyi/newmedicine**

4. What Is Cancer?

1. Amici di Dirk. (2022b, *September 29). Scientific Chart of Germanic New Medicine - Amici di Dirk.* Amici Di Dirk. **tht.fyi/scientificchart**

2. *Why Do Alcoholics Eat So Little? - Abbeycare.* (n.d.-c). Abbeycare. **tht.fyi/alcoholics**

3. *Sub-Saharan Africa.* (n.d.). The Cancer Atlas. **tht.fyi/cancerafrica**

4. Sakai, T., Özkurt, E., DeSantis, S., Wong, S. M., Rosenbaum, L., Zheng, H., & Golshan, M. (2019). National trends of synchronous bilateral breast cancer incidence in the United States. *Breast Cancer Research and Treatment, 178*(1), 161–167. National Library of Medicine. **tht.fyi/bilateralbreast**

5. Campobasso, D., Ferretti, S., & Frattini, A. (2017). Synchronous bilateral testis cancer: clinical and oncological management. *Wspolczesna Onkologia-Contemporary Oncology,* 1, 70–76. National Library of Medicine. **tht.fyi/bilateraltestis**

5. Why a Terminal Cancer Diagnosis Is Incorrect

1. *Phantom Limb Pain: What is It, Causes, Treatment & Outcome.* (n.d.). Cleveland Clinic. **tht.fyi/cleveland**

2. *Siemens on artefacts in CT scans | Germanische (Germanic) Heilkunde.* (n.d.). Germanische Heilkunde. **tht.fyi/artefacts**

3. *Amazon.in.* (n.d.). Amazon. **tht.fyi/inka**

6. Switch Off Terminal Cancer Pain

1. West, M. (2021, July 29). *What is the fight, flight, or freeze response?* Medical News Today. **tht.fyi/fightflight**

7. The Realities of Cancer Research

1. *Health Nut News.* (n.d.). Health Nut News. **tht.fyi/healthnutnews**

2. *The German/Germanic New Medicine.* (n.d.). The German New Medicine. **tht.fyi/newmedicine**

3. Pilhar, H. (2020, October 16). *Marc Fréchet - Gericht Köln Zeugenaussage - Germanische Heilkunde.* Akademie Für Germanische Heilkunde. **tht.fyi/marcfrechet**

4. *Brustkrebs, der häufigste Krebs bei Frauen Germanische Heilkunde.* (2021, January 24). Akademie Für Germanische Heilkunde. **tht.fyi/breastcancer**

5. Pilhar, H. (2020b, October 16). *Marc Fréchet - Nachruf von Dr. Hamer - Germanische Heilkunde.* Akademie Für Germanische Heilkunde. **tht.fyi/obituary**

6. Morgan, G., Ward, R., & Barton, M. (2004). *The Contribution of Cytotoxic Chemotherapy to 5-year Survival in Adult Malignancies.* The Royal College of Radiologists. **tht.fyi/chemostudy**

7. Gøtzsche, P. C. (2014). *Our prescription drugs kill us in large numbers. Polskie Archiwum Medycyny Wewnetrznej-Polish Archives of Internal Medicine.* National Library of Medicine. **tht.fyi/pubmed3rdleadingcause**

8. *Study Suggests Medical Errors Now Third Leading Cause of Death in the U.S. - 05/03/2016.* (n.d.-b). Johns Hopkins Medicine. **tht.fyi/hopkins3rdleadingcause**

8. Healing with Music Therapy

1. *Fibonacci in Music, Fibonacci.* (2019, April 17). Fibonacci. **tht.fyi/fibonacci**

2. *Verdi Tuning - brief history.* (n.d.). The Schiller Institute. **tht.fyi/schiller**

3. Amici di Dirk. (2022a, February 3). *Video Presentation on Mein Studentenmädchen - Amici di Dirk.* Amici Di Dirk. **tht.fyi/healingmusic**

4. Amici di Dirk. (n.d.). *Audio-Cd Archives - Amici di Dirk.* Amici Di Dirk. **tht.fyi/purchasehealingmusic**

9. Learn GHk/GNM to Help Yourself and Others

1. Herbs and Health Holistic Center. (n.d.). *Books.* GNM Online Seminars. **tht.fyi/gnmproducts**

2. *What's German New Medicine?* (n.d.-b). Andi Locke Mears. **tht.fyi/andilockemears**

3. *What is Germanische Heilkunde?* (n.d.). GHK Pilhar Academy. **tht.fyi/pilharacademy**

4. *GNM Institute.* (n.d.). GNM Institute. **tht.fyi/gnminstitute**

5. *Resources - Danny Carroll.* (2023, March 6). Danny Carroll. **tht.fyi/resources**

ABOUT THE AUTHOR

Danny spent the first half of his life living in London, UK, and completed his education with a master's degree from the London School of Economics. He moved to live and work in India in the mid-1990s.

Danny has spent the last seventeen years studying alternative healing therapies in search of the Holy Grail of health and wellness. Following a cathartic healing experience in 2012, he has focused on mind-body healing protocols for the last ten years. He discovered a new body of medical knowledge called Germanic Healing Knowledge (GHk), or Germanic New Medicine (GNM), developed by a German medical doctor named Ryke Geerd Hamer. He has spent the last seven years using this medical science to help people with chronic and terminal health conditions to fully recover their health.

"Terminal Cancer Is a Misdiagnosis" is Danny's first book. He plans to write a 500+ series of books examining how Conventional Medicine and Germanic Healing Knowledge approach the cause, symptoms, and solutions to specific diseases. Danny is a pioneer of new medical discoveries and healing protocols that most are unwilling to explore, until they have no other alternative.

Email: dc@danny-carroll.com
Website: danny-carroll.com

 facebook.com/thehealingtribune

 pinterest.com/thehealingtribune

Manufactured by Amazon.ca
Acheson, AB

11713006R00046